CONFESSIONS

OF

BUTTERFLIES

Hidden Truths of Living in Pain

Joanna Dwyer

DEDICATION

To My "Fibro Fighters":

I didn't write this text. You did. My support system; my team, the people who go through this painful journey with me day in and day out.

This is a collection of your voices – your struggles and triumphs – and I hope I did it right. This book wouldn't exist without your raw and candid words, and it would be awfully hard for me to exist without all of you.

Thank you from the deepest depths of my heart and soul and never stop fighting. This is for you.

To my cheerleader, my coach, and my friend, Des.

Without you, I would still be tearing my hair out over chapter two. You dragged me through it, kicking and screaming, until this shattered mess turned into something worth reading.

CONTENTS

INTRODUCTION

This is for the people who suffer in silence. The people who work, raise children, care for their parents, cook and clean, teach and sacrifice every moment of every day despite being in constant, unrelenting, unforgiving pain.

This is our voice. The voice of the "too young." The ones who get passed from doctor to doctor, who get belittled by family. The ones who get left by their partner, who grieve their previous life, who ache with guilt and wrestle with wanting to die but needing to live.

This is our truth. This is the stuff you don't want to hear because it is ugly and it is raw, and, worst of all, there's nothing you can do about it.

We are tired of screaming in silence and sick of the snide comments, the unwanted advice and the rolling eyes. We are not who you think we are. We are not lying, helpless, or needy. We are not weak. We are not old and frail. We are young, and we are sick.

We have become so used to hiding that we have forgotten we are valuable. We save our tears for the middle of the night, for quiet moments in between work and home, for showers and bed. We can't see how strong we are, because we leave no weakness for comparison.

Because of that, we have built an underground network of support groups where we are free to scream and cry, wail and say "fuck you" to the world fearlessly and honestly. We're free to break down, show our scars, bleed our pain, and ask for help. Our groups are a solace in a world that widely ignores us. Every day one of us thanks the group for saving their life.

Every so often someone new will join. She will be broken, exhausted, on the verge of giving up, desperate for someone – anyone – to listen and understand, even for one minute.

And we do. We understand.

When I asked my support group what they would want the world to know, the one thing they'd want to say, they replied;

Believe us.

That's all. We just want to be believed. Trust me, we are hard enough on ourselves. No one could possibly be more critical and hateful of ourselves than us. Having someone believe, even just one person, could mean the world.

If you are living in chronic pain, I hope this book is your voice. I hope I can say what you need the world to hear. And I hope you find comfort in knowing that you are far from alone.

If you don't have chronic pain, I hope this book helps you believe. Whether you know someone with chronic pain or not, if you think it's all a scam or just in our heads, I hope this book changes how you see us.

Why the butterfly?

The butterfly is the symbol for fibromyalgia. I'm not sure how this came to be, but it makes sense. The Butterfly Effect, which stems from the Chaos theory, tells us that something, no matter how small or quiet, can change the world. That the tiny force of flapping wings can cause a tornado halfway across the globe.

The butterfly is us, the pain warriors, those who hurt silently and live our days enduring rather than living. We do have an effect on the world. We have a presence, a purpose, and we deserve to be acknowledged.

If we speak up, we will be heard. If we flap our wings, our wind will be felt.

We do matter, and this book is our butterfly effect.

.

I didn't ask for this and believe me, I don't want it. I know you roll your eyes, even when you try and hide it. I know you think I'm exaggerating or being dramatic. But this is something I wouldn't wish on anyone.

You're used to seeing me work and cook, clean and go shopping, and go out with friends. I don't complain often because if I did every time I was in pain, I would have nothing else to say. If I'm complaining, just know it must be really severe.

The truth is, I'm living a double life.

I do all these things with a smile on my face because I have no choice. The only other option would be to wallow in bed and watch life pass me by.

You see me take my pain meds and wonder if I'm addicted. I take my pain meds and wonder how I will function if they are taken from me. I don't get high, I get normal. I take those meds to feel better as you take yours when you have a cold. They are the reason I can do all the other things you see me doing every day.

The truth is, I'm sick of the relentless pain. I cry when you're not looking. I wake up in the night writhing in pain while you're sleeping. I clench my teeth when you ask me to do something physical while you don't even give it a second thought. I do 100 things a day that you don't notice because I hide it. I hide my pain, I hide my fatigue, I hide my guilt and frustration.

The truth is, I watch you and wonder what it's like to feel like that – to be able to do all these things without pain and fatigue. I want to break down and scream and cry. I get so angry I want to smash everything around me.

I wonder if I can keep going like this.

But the part that's worse than the pain? Knowing you don't believe me. That no matter how much I try and tell you, you won't understand. So I keep it to myself.

Even when I'm surrounded by people, I'm still alone with my pain.

I'm not helpless. I don't want you to feel bad for me. I don't want special treatment.

All I want is some empathy.

Don't get mad at me when I can't do something. Don't get frustrated when I can't go somewhere. Don't judge me when I take my meds. Don't call me lazy when I sleep more often, especially since I haven't slept the past four nights.

Please just don't make me feel guilty for having this disease.

Just try and believe me. That's all I want.

Love,

A Girl with Chronic Pain

OUR DARK PASSENGER

Chronic pain is invisible. People can't see our pain or how hard we try to overcome our symptoms.

We smile more, laugh more, work more, push more. But there is a dark side to chronic pain, a side most of us will never talk about. We can't talk about these things with "regular" people ("normies".) We are afraid to mention it to our doctors in fear of being institutionalized or losing our medications because we have been labeled "addiction risk."

So I'll just say it.

Some days when I think about the fact that I have felt like this for over a decade, and will continue for many decades to come, I wonder if life is worth living. And I am not alone.

So many people – parents, children, spouses, caregivers, teachers, students, mentors – feel the exact same way.

Not only is chronic pain highly stigmatized, so are depression and suicide. It is safer to keep it to ourselves. Discussions are filled with statements like "I would never actually do it but..." Recently a woman posted in a fibromyalgia group, "I would never touch heroin, but sometimes *I just want to inject myself to take the pain and depression away.*"

My heart dropped because I was afraid for her, afraid that people would respond negatively and put her down for her feelings. But, to my surprise, her post led to a long string of resounding understanding and agreement. Women began to not only admit to fantasizing about trying heroin, but also to suicidal feelings.

It was the most powerful, liberating conversation I have ever seen. Screw the stigma, they cried, and let's talk about this.

How incredible.

A woman recently asked the group if having children made fibromyalgia worse. Again the overwhelming and honest responses began to flow. My chest nearly burst with joy as I read through everyone's comments. So many moms candidly talking about their feelings of depression, anxiety and suicide. I am not alone! Yet every mother's answer also stated that their kids save their lives every day, becoming the reason they push through and cope.

That is when I realized their stories are also my own.

Every morning I wake up with stiff muscles on fire, joints stabbing me, exhausted no matter how much I slept. I wake up knowing that I have to get through another day.

I wake up feeling like I don't want to wake up anymore.

But then my children burst into my bedroom, thrilled to see me. They hug me and kiss me and wish me a good morning, and their warmth soothes the agony in my mind. I forget about my incessant pain, the endless fatigue and the frustration of my poor cognition.

I get up for them. I go to work for them. I come home for them. I agree to carry on for them. My children save me from myself and I belong to them, not to my disease.

My story is not unique. There are millions of me.

We battle our bodies for the people in our lives. We choose to live. We accept this sadness, this daunting condition, this bottomless depression so we can live for other people. Because when you have fibromyalgia, or any invisible illness, you have to decide every day whether to end the pain now or endure the suffering for a lifetime.

We choose to battle ourselves and keep smiling in the darkness. Every time we choose life, we deserve to speak openly and vent honestly without fear, without shame and without stigmatization.

We are warriors and our fight should not be a secret.

Without our voices, fibromyalgia and chronic pain will remain invisible.

In the show Dexter, the main character has an alter–ego living inside of him. He calls it his "dark passenger" because he can't get rid of it or tell anyone about it, he has to just keep living with it.

He lives an apparently normal life. Work, friends, family, marriage, etc, but at the end of the day, it's just him and his dark passenger. He has to come to terms with the fact that it's not going anywhere and he can't ignore it. He has to accept and make life work with it.

While us butterflies aren't serial killers, though if we were, we would be good ones like Dexter. We have our own dark passenger.

"I feel trapped by this body. I feel much bigger than it will let me be. Sometimes it feels as though I'm breathing with glass in my lungs. My bones feel bruised and throbbing. It's distracting, it taints many moments, steals them." — Tiara W.

Our pain is invisible, and it is always present. While in the beginning we might fight like hell, desperate to rid ourselves of this monster, we eventually realize there is no way. We have to accept it.

"I feel as if there's tiny monsters eating my bones. They're gnawing at the core of my bones and it feels as if they may give at any time. I can feel their sharp fangs and claws digging into my bones." — Aurora G.

So, like our dear friend Dexter, we live a double–life. There is the life that you see; working, going out, shopping, cooking, cleaning, laughing like nothing is wrong. and the life we hide. Because when you're not looking, when we have you fooled, our dark passenger comes out to play.

As you read each paragraph in this book, you wouldn't know how long it took me to write. I had to get up and walk around every five or ten minutes because the stabbing, aching and burning in my body became unbearable. At times my computer lay dormant for weeks because my pain flared and I couldn't concentrate on anything for longer than a minute. Sometimes I stopped writing out of fear that nobody would even care enough to pick this book up.

No one knew that struggle but me because I never let anyone see it.

Our dark passenger is with us all day, every day, and you would never know. We have become adept actors, working twice as hard to appear normal, figuring out how to get through each minute of each day, every day.

We butterflies don't want anyone to have to deal with our pain. We feel like a burden to ourselves already, so we go above and beyond to keep from being one to everyone around us. That is why some butterflies become so desperate they take their own life.

By the average pain scale, we live anywhere from a five to an eight. This would usually send someone to the urgent clinic. We take our meds and keep going.

Know that if you do hear a butterfly complaining about pain, they mean it. We usually won't until we're well above an eight.

My boss doesn't know that it takes me a good hour to get from the bed to the car because my body needs time to loosen up and for my pain meds sink in. My clients don't know that I broke down crying twice while grooming their dog because pain shocked my body during.

I have a very physically demanding job. I am a dog groomer. I bend, I stand on my feet eight to ten hours a day, I wrestle and lift 100 pound dogs. My upper body doesn't get a rest, and my arms are in constant motion.

I have worked during early labor, four herniated discs, tendinitis, and a permanent shoulder injury, yet none of those compare to the pain of working with a fibromyalgia flare. But I am not special and I am not unique.

We do this every day.

We choose to work, to bear children, to cook and clean, to take on endeavors that we really shouldn't, all in the name of being normal. The other choice is to lay in bed, avoid life, and depend on everyone else for everything. No, thanks. We will save that for last.

This doesn't mean we don't have moments of weakness where we give in to the grief and hopelessness. Of course we do. The dark passenger is always there, always ready to take hold of our minds and hearts in an instant, and we fight. Hard. Always.

That is when we reach out to the people who will get it, and they help us through the night so we can go back to life the next morning, no one else knowing what hell we had been in the night before.

Our battles are endless and complex. We have to prove ourselves day in and day out to family, coworkers, doctors and so on. We fight for our lives every moment.

Every morning when we wake up, we lay there and ask ourselves if we can go on. Is this worth getting out of bed for? Am I tired enough yet? Am I ready to give in?

Then we think of our children. Our partner. Our parents. Our pets. They fuel our determination to not let the disease win, at least that day.

"I didn't ask for this disease and all its accompanying conditions, but I can't let it define and rule my life either. I push through every single day because I don't have a choice. I have three sets of eyes looking to me to provide them with a childhood they don't have to recover from...being bedridden isn't an option. Don't get me wrong, I don't think any less of someone who is bedridden, I know it's not their choice. I just know I can't. Even when the pain gets really bad I

push through for them. For my children who did not ask to have a sick mom. They deserve the best I can give and I'll be damned if I don't try my hardest, my very best, to be the kind of mom they deserve." — Sarah R.

At the end of the day, when we are finally alone with our pain, our dark passenger, only then do we give ourselves permission to collapse under the weight of it all.

Then we wake up the next morning and began anew.

CONFESSIONS

The only people privy to the realities of our life are other sick people. We've been trained to stay silent, to smile, to fake it for the sake of everyone around us. We confess to one another because it is safe.

I want to share some of those "confessions" with you. If you don't have chronic pain, I hope these words help you understand what we feel. I asked every butterfly I know to explain their pain as if they're talking only to us; not how they explain it to their doctors or family or co-workers – the sugar-coated version – I wanted the real, raw, ugly truth.

If you do have chronic pain, I hope these confessions make you feel less alone, less crazy, and less scared. We are all in this together and yes, we get it.

"It feels like my muscles are being pulled from my bones. Remember the growing pains you got growing up? Imagine waking up one day to never–ending growing pains turned up to the max. It's living with the ache of a fever, even when your temp is low. It's migraines out of nowhere because the sun is just a little bit too bright that day. It's fingers that randomly decide not to work, toes that go numb for no reason, and elbows that ache just from holding your phone too long. It's hips and knees that feel like they're grinding together when there's no evidence of that happening.

But that's just the physical stuff. There's also the social and emotional impact of it. Who wants to invite someone out when they always say no because they're too tired/sick/ouchy? People tend to just give up on you and it can make it difficult not to give up on yourself. It's depression setting in even when things look great on the outside because who can feel this way and not feel at least a little bit sorry for themselves? It's anxiety keeping you from going out to the zoo or museum because, more than likely, that trip will be very painful.

It's the fear of going to the doctor or ER because even when you know that the problem isn't caused by fibro, you also know that more than likely you'll have to fight with the doctor to even get them to do any tests. It's the exhaustion not just from the pain, but from all of the emotional labor, including the labor of constantly fighting for yourself.

But it isn't all bad. It gives you a completely new perspective. It helps you understand and empathize so much better. It gives you new language and a better way to speak to other chronically ill people or even just struggling people. IT gives you a strength that you didn't know that you were ever capable of having because even if your body is weak, you're fighting every damn day.

Sometimes you have to take a break and let yourself be weak, but if you don't pick yourself up and get back to struggling and fighting your way through, you'll have no life. So all of a sudden, you realize that you've learned to fight for yourself. You've learned that you can stand up for yourself and put yourself first, even when it seems impossible.

You can fight through the pain and exhaustion to take those trips and have the most fulfilling life you can.

It's having to look on the bright side, because if you let yourself get sucked into that hole of self–pity and depression, it can take a miracle and a ton of work to drag yourself out. And it's also knowing that you'll end up in that hole sometimes, so having a support system in place is probably the single most important thing you can do for yourself." — Richelle R.

ON PARENTING AND PARTNERSHIP

When you have chronic pain, it affects everyone you are close to. While everyone responds differently to our disease, there is a common thread in every relationship a butterfly has and that is guilt. We are programmed to believe we have to be a certain kind of wife, mother, and child. If we don't meet those expectations, we are failures. This has to stop. We are just as worthy as a healthy person. We didn't ask to be sick, and we push ourselves every day far past what our body is capable of, for the sake of others.

We need to realize that our families love us for who we are, not for what we can do.

FIBRO GUILT: PARENTING WITH PAIN

"Mommy, do you want to come on a walk with us?" My daughter asks me this every time her dad takes them on a nature hike. And every time my answer is no. She knows I won't go but I suppose she asks just in case one day I'll say yes. So off they will go with flashlights and jars to catch lightning bugs, leaving me on the couch with my guilt and pain medication, feeling the weight of guilt on my chest.

Guilt goes hand in hand with fibromyalgia, especially if you're a parent. Missing out on so many of your kids' activities is heartbreaking and can be overwhelming.

You feel guilty for missing out on playtime, you feel guilty for being crabby, you feel guilty for getting them to school late because your medication makes you groggy in the morning and every day is a new experience in what you couldn't do.

Ask anyone with fibro and they will tell you that they are constantly apologizing to at least one person in their life. Whether to children, parents, partners, or friends, guilt might as well be classified as a symptom.

I frequently decline invitations to dinner, movies, hanging out, etc., and then spend a large amount of my time apologizing to them for it.

But I apologize the most to my children.

I am sorry I can't go on walks with you. I'm sorry we didn't go to your friends' birthday party because I wasn't feeling well and daddy was at work.

Children are naturally compassionate little people and surprisingly have a good grasp on an illness they can't even pronounce yet. When my kids want to lay on me they now know to ask "Mommy, does this hurt you?" When I'm moving slowly they ask "Mommy, does your body hurt a lot today?"

It brings tears to my eyes when they have to ask those questions. I wish they could flop into my arms without worry. I desperately want to do all the mom things I feel I'm supposed to, like cuddles and hikes and birthday parties.

As hard as it may be, you have to remind yourself that it is not your fault. You should not apologize for something that is out of your control. When you explain your illness to your kids, you are not making excuses.. But a mother will do anything to protect her children from pain, emotional and physical, and I feel like I am hurting them when I have to opt out of activities or ask them to stop touching me because it's too painful.

What kind of a mother does that?

We do.

We have to.

I remind myself that I have raised intelligent, compassionate, resilient little humans who get everything from me that I can give. Between their father and me, they get all the love they need.

When they're adults, they're not going to remember mom missing out on nature walks, they will remember how loved they were.

I am not damaging them, but my guilt is damaging me and I have to learn to let go of it. All a mother can do is the best she can with what she's got, and we've got a lot of love to give.

PARENTING IN THE FOG

Can you imagine a parent forgetting to register their child for school? Because I have done that.

I forget not just my own commitments, but my kids, and I get angry with myself over it. What kind of a mother doesn't pack an afternoon snack for her kid to bring to school? What kind of a mother misses entire days worth of antibiotic doses?

What kind of mother sees that her children's rooms are in shambles but does nothing about it? I'll tell you who. A mother with fibromyalgia.

I am a very disorganized person. I make lists, then forget them. I make appointments, then miss them. I have two calendars, but can never remember to use them. I am in a constant state of brain fog, affectionately known as Fibro Fog to us.

While I'm sure this is an incredibly frustrating thing for everyone dealing with it, it is exceptionally tricky for parents and caregivers. It is more than annoying, it is embarrassing and scary.

People tend to look down on messy houses and skipped commitments much more when it involves children. I take extra care to try and remember, especially for my kids, but a lot of the times it just doesn't happen and I am constantly afraid of the consequences. I have been scolded for forgetting things like buying my daughter new shoes, and been called careless and self–absorbed because I forgot such basic things.

I'm not. I just forgot.

I want to scream this at her and everyone else who accuses me of being careless or lazy. I forget everything all the time and feel awful, I don't need others to make me feel even worse.

Not only are my children perpetually late for everything, but it is guaranteed that they are missing something whether it be a snack or a permission slip. My seven year old keeps better track of her due dates and school functions than I do. But forgetting school stuff isn't even the worst of it.

I forgot to give my son his antibiotics for three days in a row. When I did remember, the anxiety set in. What if he gets sicker? *I'll have to tell the doctor I forgot his meds, then the doctor will call child services on me. Oh god what have I done?!* My son is fine; perfectly healthy.

Don't we all forget to take our full round of antibiotics anyway? But it's different when it's a child.

I am afraid of being judged by other parents and by their teachers. I am afraid of a doctor saying something is wrong because of my neglect. I am afraid of my kids getting left out or teased because of me. I am afraid of someone coming over and telling other people "you won't believe how messy her house is – I can't believe she has kids!"

But so far in my seven years of momming none of these terrible things have happened and my kids are all but unaffected by my foggy brain. We have learned to laugh things off for the most part.

My husband is in charge of keeping track of everything. My keys, my doctor's appointments, what day it is, and what planet we're on, etc. There have been a few monumental screw-ups on my part, like when I forgot my daughter's dress rehearsal for the ballet recital she had prepared for all year. She wasn't allowed to be in the performance because of it. My daughter was over it in a matter of hours but I spent the better part of a week verbally assaulting myself over it.

I've forgotten to pay bills resulting in a shut-off notice and forget birthdays on a regular basis.

I'm a mess.

But I am training myself to stop abusing myself because of it.

Like everything else that is a result of fibromyalgia, this is not my fault. I am learning to be more open and honest about how my brain works (or doesn't, I should say). I set alarms with notes to myself to remind me, and pass information along to my husband immediately before I forget. As someone who loses her glasses ten times a day and wanders around the house aimlessly should not be in charge of anything important.

Since I've let go of the pressure of doing it all myself, we've found a good balance and the missed appointments and forgotten performances have gone down to a bare minimum. When I do forget something, it's not the end of the world. No one has the right to judge me if they aren't living the life I have. My house isn't messy, it's lived in. And my children are not going to be ruined because I forgot a classmate's birthday party. Kids won't remember little things like these, but they will remember a mother who constantly beats herself up, so that is the behavior that has to stop.

PAINKILLERS AND PARENTING

When I first began seeing doctors for my condition, they gave me Tylenol–3 with Codeine. For the first time in a long time, I felt good. The pills brought the pain down from an 8 to a 3. I remember putting on my running shoes and going outside and taking a short jog around the block. But my joy was short–lived as the judgment began.

The stigma around opioids is growing.

People lump heroin and prescription opioids together, and equate heroin addicts and responsible patients taking prescribed medications.

Inevitably came the question, "How can you take care of your kids when you're on pain killers?"

What kind of question is that?

I wondered why this person felt entitled to ask me something so personal and if she would ask the same question if I were taking blood pressure medication? For a moment I felt like a criminal, but then a wave of confidence came over me. I wasn't going to shrug it off anymore. I decided to call her out.

"Actually, without these meds I wouldn't be able to care for my children at all. I'm a much more functional parent with them, that's why my doctor prescribes them. Please don't conflate my pain with addiction."

My parenting improved with pain medication. I could actually move my body without excruciating pain, which meant I was in a positive mind–state and and could play and bond with my children. I was happy

People don't realize how much chronic pain can affect your life beyond the physical symptoms.

Chronic pain makes you tired, depressed, anxious, angry, and frustrated.

Before pain medication, I spent most of my time in a bad mood. I would snap at my husband and kids. I could not tolerate loud sounds, even the sound of my kids' voices were like nails on a chalkboard. I would literally have a physical reaction like an electric storm to some sounds. At one point my daughter asked me; "Mommy, why are you angry all the time?"

That question hurt far more than any question about my parenting with pills.

Yet I began to wonder, is it bad parenting to take opioids? Does it affect my parenting? Is it as the same as being drunk or high?

I began to judge myself when I took a pill in front of my kids. I felt ashamed for taking my own prescription medication. I would sometimes not take it to see if I was a "better mom" without my meds. I felt like a drug addict. And I was completely miserable.

Without pills, I could barely move around and stewed in the darkest, angriest of moods. Not because I needed a fix, but because my body depended on prescription medication to function as close to normally as it can get.

Then I realized that there is a difference between addiction and dependence.

Would someone tell a mother who takes insulin that her medication makes her a reckless parent? Absolutely not, because her life depends on it. Ironically, however, there is an entire "mom culture" centered on drinking wine while parenting which people laugh about and raise their glass to.

Why is it okay to rain down judgment on a pain patient? I am prescribed Tramadol for a reason and that reason is to improve my quality of life. I am able to function like a normal, happy, energetic and attentive mother when I take my meds. Without them I am an angry zombie.

When I tried my no–med experiment, my husband saw the agony I dealt with; an invisible illness becoming visible. He knew why I tried not to take my opioids, to prove the judge and jury wrong. When he couldn't take it anymore, he gently said, "Joanna, just take your meds. You don't have to prove anything to anyone. Your doctor gave them to you for a reason."

I asked him what prompted that, and he responded, "Because I can see you're in pain and struggling...and you're really hard to be around when you're in pain," he added with a chuckle.

I had my "proof." I am a happier, more functional person when I take my opioids regularly. And you know what? It is not open for public comment.

No one has the right to judge me based on societal stigmas, especially not someone who doesn't suffer through chronic pain. You think parenting is hard? Try doing it when your body feels like it has been flattened by an elephant then set on fire, then talk to me, talk to any of us, about our struggles.

MY HUSBAND IS THE "BETTER" PARENT (AND I'M OK WITH THAT)

As I sat at dinner with my children one night, my daughter asked me something profound. "Mommy, how come Daddy does everything for us and you don't?" My jaw dropped. I didn't know how to react or respond.

"What does Daddy do?" I asked.

"He cleans the house and makes us dinner. He takes us to school. He takes us places like on nature walks and the park and bike rides."

"And what does Mommy do?" I asked.

She thought for a minute then responded: "You go to work and you come home and lay on the couch."

I wasn't angry, or upset, because it's true.

For the past year my husband has been the one doing all the parenting activities that are normally done by the mom. You know, the things that moms are always complaining about being underappreciated for and writing top ten lists about and wishing their husbands would help with.

I have always been a workhorse, and still am, but last October I went on a medical leave for five months due to what I now know is Fibromyalgia. I spent my days on the couch unable to cook, clean or do pretty much anything. It was the first time in my adult life I couldn't work.

The pain prevented me from doing all the things that come natural to me as a hard–worker, a mother, and wife. I became overwhelmingly depressed and my kids and husband were left to carry on without me. He picked up my slack with no complaint, all while working nights managing a bar. He kept the kids at bay when I was having hard days and made sure they were dressed, fed, and homework done.

He took them out on adventures after school so I could have more quiet time, as he knew I was sensitive to sound, including my own kids' voices.

My depression got even worse as I began to feel like a bum mother.

What was wrong with me? Why couldn't I just do all the "mom things" I wanted to?

I judged myself harshly and beat myself up constantly over my inability to care for my children, my home and my husband. I felt I should have been the one taking them to the park and making their breakfast in the morning. These were my way of contributing and bonding with my kids. If I wasn't helping my son brush his teeth in the morning then what was my role? I felt lost and displaced.

Without realizing it, I had distanced myself from my family out of self–loathing and disappointment. I began lashing out at my husband, picking fights with him for reasons I can't even remember now. It was out of anger and frustration with myself and envy for my husband's abilities and strong relationship with our children.

I resented him for being the better parent.

I apologized a lot, but never to myself. I apologized to my husband and children, who were so kind and understanding it made me feel even worse. My husband supported me and was perfectly content to assume both roles in our household.

When my daughter asked me that question, I asked her how she felt about it. Her response was simple. "I don't mind."

That's when it dawned on me that my kids didn't see it as "mommy's job" and "daddy's job." They don't care which one of us it is taking them on nature walks or dropping them off at school, they just want us to be happy parents. I realized they were bonding more with my husband not because he was the better parent, but because he exuded happiness.

He spent time with them and all kids really need or want is your time. And I was wasting it wallowing in my self–pity and anger over my disease. My kids saw me unhappy, depressed, and resentful of their father. I was toxic.

That's when I decided that even though I couldn't go on a five–mile bike ride, hiking in the woods, or even wake up early didn't mean that I couldn't participate in my kids' life. Or my own.

I sat down and explained to them Fibromyalgia as simply as I could. I told them that although I couldn't do all the things that Daddy does, we could still do things together, like homework, art projects, and reading. They excitedly began rattling off ideas of things we could do together and relief swept over me.

I finally went back to work, which helped with my self–esteem, and gave me back a feeling of contribution to the household. My husband still does the majority of the parenting, only now I've realized he does it because he wants to – because he loves me and loves our kids. He understands what I need and his abilities as a father do not take away from mine, they compensate for the abilities I don't have. I realize just how lucky I am to have a partner who truly believes and understands me.

HE DIDN'T ASK FOR THIS

My husband didn't ask for Fibromyalgia, but he experiences aspects of it every day. No, he doesn't understand my pain, but he doesn't pretend to either.

Guilt is one of the worst symptoms of chronic pain, I have yet to meet a fellow butterfly who isn't carrying around the weight of guilt at all times, apologizing incessantly and unnecessarily.

We often feel like a burden and spend most of our energy, what little we have, trying to make up for it without realizing that the other person is choosing to be with us. Sure, sometimes he rolls his eyes at me and once or twice he's said, "There's *always something wrong with you!*" I used to take these things personally until I looked at it from his perspective.

How would I feel if my husband who was once "normal" became increasingly sick and unable to function? If we no longer went places and did things we used to and I had to make up for all the things he could no longer do? Yeah, I would probably get frustrated from time to time.

I began to make it a point to thank him whenever I could and to push myself harder to do things for him. I used to say "no" to every single thing he wanted to do until eventually he stopped asking. Now, I take a little extra time to prepare physically and emotionally, and I go.

Not only does this make him happy, it usually makes me feel pretty good too, because I've accomplished something for our marriage.

Intimacy is another aspect of our relationship that he probably didn't expect to be giving up before we even hit thirty years old. I could go weeks, even months, without having sex and to be honest, for a long time that's exactly what I did. My husband never complained, never pressured me, but it dawned on me that for most people, sex is a routine part of intimacy, and I had withdrawn it without acknowledging his feelings.

He knows I do the best I can, but I want to make him feel good as well. So, like with everything else, I prepare myself physically and mentally beforehand and I'm usually pleased after.

Having a physical connection to your partner does wonders for your relationship and for yourself. Satisfaction can come in many forms, and I hadn't realized how much I missed the emotional intimacy that comes with it.

We've found other ways to be intimate, ways that are more comfortable for me. Honestly, we've had to do that in every aspect of our partnership. While thinking about writing this section, I decided to get some "confessions" directly from him.

"Husband, what's it like being married to me? What do you struggle with? What are your biggest frustrations? Do you ever wish your wife was normal?"

I was prepared for him to rattle off a long list of things he hates about my disease and how much he's given up for me. He said this instead:

"It is what it is. I just have to deal with it. I'm lucky because I don't have to go through it [fibromyalgia]."

All I could do was hug him.

We get so wrapped up in this disease, the pain can often blind us to the struggles of our partner, family, or anyone we share a life with. A little "thank you" can go a long way.

We can't forget to appreciate the ones who support us unconditionally.

"BUT YOU DON'T LOOK SICK"

People with fibromyalgia are incredible actors.

Most people would never guess we're sick. In fact, we're so good at pretending to be normal that when we do admit to our disease, people flat–out don't believe us. Most of us are so sick of the disbelief we don't even bother telling people anymore. It goes something like this:

"I have fibromyalgia."

"Really? But you don't look sick!" (Translation; I don't believe you.)

"Oh, yeah. My grandma has that." (Translation; you're too young.)

"I've heard that pain comes from stress." (Translation; it's all in your head.)

And don't get me started on doctors. Yes, doctors. Sometimes they're worse than everyone else.

Let's be honest, when you think of someone with fibromyalgia, or any other chronic pain disease, you probably don't imagine someone under the age of fifty. That is due to the stigmas surrounding chronic pain, and the lack of research and general knowledge.

People expect older people to be sick, whether they look it or not, and no one is surprised to discover they are. But take someone like me, a thirty–three year old mother of two, working, writing, running a household, and you wouldn't believe how many times I hear, "Wow, I had no idea!" As if I am some sort of magician and just gave away my secret.

But I know what that means. What they really want to say to me is; "That's funny, you don't look sick and if you were, how could you do all those things?"

Because I have to.

Most healthy people know as much about fibromyalgia as a Lyrica commercial tells them. The list of symptoms flow through the background, minimizing the effects on the viewer's mind. Widespread pain and fatigue? That doesn't sound so bad. The characters in the commercials are older and often depicted struggling to do simple daily hobbies like gardening.

No wonder nobody thinks we're sick.

A more accurate picture would be a worn–down mother, lying awake in her bed crying, then dragging herself from bed to car to work, faking smiles and hiding her struggle every ten minutes to get through the day. Or a retail employee sleeping in the breakroom, unable to face the over–stimulation of the store. Or even a college student writing an email to her professor explaining why she hasn't been in class the last week and begging for time to get caught up.

"You don't look sick" is a sugarcoated way of saying "I don't believe you." and we know it.

We know we don't "look" sick.

We know we are "too young" and we know you see us doing everything we do each day, but that doesn't mean you know the battle within our bodies.

WORKING WITH FIBRO

Since being diagnosed with Fibromyalgia, I've spent a lot of time in online support groups. You can vent and speak freely, and find hundreds of others who know exactly what you are going through. These groups have been a lifesaver for me, often literally

People in group often ask questions like "What do you think this pain could be?" and "Does anyone use any natural supplements for fatigue?" and so on. But there is one question that I see pop up frequently that brings a rush of anger and despair every time I see it. "Should I tell my new employer that I have Fibromyalgia?"

The fact that anyone has to ask that is wrong in so many ways. First off, it is illegal for an employer to discriminate against anyone for a medical reason or disability. Secondly, why do we feel so much fear about our condition? The people asking this question are afraid of being treated differently, losing hours, promotions, and even losing their job altogether. And to be honest, I was one of those people.

Last year my rotator cuff tore, which resulted in tendinitis, that I had to go on a medical leave for. I am a dog groomer, and without a right shoulder it is impossible to do my job. I was gone for months and as my time off piled up, I began to worry that I would going to be replaced even though my job is protected by FMLA (Family Medical Leave Act).

When the doctor told me that I had Fibromyalgia, I felt terrified. I was the manager of an extremely busy grooming salon, and had an incredible amount of pressure on me. I was also working toward a promotion.

How would Fibromyalgia affect that?

I sat down in the office with my boss, who was a wonderful manager and a better mentor. My hands shook and I could feel tears stinging my eyes as I fumbled for the words to tell him about my diagnosis. I had played out the scene in my head of me telling him and him saying that my career was over.

When I finally spit it out, he looked at me and said, *"Well, that's good news! You can handle that! It could have been much worse. Just make sure to take care of yourself."*

I was so relieved I felt like I melted.

When I moved out of state and transferred to a new salon, I felt confident enough to tell my new boss upfront that I have Fibromyalgia, and explained how it can affect me at work sometimes, but that I have learned how to work with it. He was also supportive and has never once brought up my condition or used it against me.

However, as I scroll through my support groups and read these gut–wrenching stories about people's hours getting cut and losing their jobs I want to scream. I want to march into their office and shake their managers.

We are not our illness. We can do it. We might forget occasionally or be sluggish some days, or need to sit down if our job requires us to stand. But we are tough and determined.

If Fibromyalgia has taught us anything it's that we have to work twice as hard as a healthy person and we are determined to prove that we can do it.

Don't doubt us.

Fibromyalgia is a challenge that we did not have a choice in. But do you know what can impede us? Stress. And do you know what is stressful? Having and maintaining a job. When we feel that our job, our source of income and often medical insurance, is being threatened, it exacerbates our symptoms.

If you put the idea in our heads that we might not have a job, we will not sleep, our pain will increase tremendously, we will be more forgetful and become more depressed. That is what you should be afraid of, boss.

Instead of making us feel threatened because you doubt our capabilities, why don't you try making us feel supported? There is nothing more motivating than that, for healthy people and sick people alike.

My boss never doubts me so I never doubt me. I feel secure enough to leave work early if my pain gets unbearable and secure enough to laugh it off when I forget something in my Fibro Fog. I also work as hard as I can for my boss and give 100%, because I want to.

Please, friends. Do not be afraid to speak up. Be open and honest, not just about your illness, but about your skills and capabilities, too. Be confident and take the challenge. Don't let your boss's doubt take hold of you. Prove them wrong. And if your boss still doubts you, it might be time to look for a new job anyway because no one, healthy or sick, can work for someone like that.

DISABILITY

Another perk of the ageism and stigmas surrounding us? Most of us get little to no help from the government.

Disability benefits seem like a myth to us. A dream that we won't reach until we have hit a certain age, when it is deemed acceptable to suffer chronic pain. So we work. What else can we do? And because we work, we look okay.

Since we can't get government assistance, but we have families to support, we have no choice. It's either do it or have nothing. We cannot let our kids, our partners, or ourselves down, and we crawl our way through work, days or nights or both, doing our best.

We get called into the office to discuss our frequent tardiness, and we are too afraid and too embarrassed to explain the never–ending fatigue that haunts us all day and often keeps us from thinking properly. We take our medications in private so as to avoid the judgmental gazes of our healthy coworkers who "would never touch Vicodin."

I never thought of myself as "disabled" because I had always been able to work. The idea of not working was foreign, and I could not imagine doing anything else. What do people do besides work? Where does the money come from? But then, I also couldn't imagine being in so much pain I couldn't work.

I didn't realize, at the start, that this journey through hell had only just begun. Once my body started breaking down, the reality that I might have to slow down or stop crept into my thoughts, my Dark Passenger whispering in my ear.

It began with a shoulder problem, then herniated cervical discs, followed by two more herniated discs in my lumbar spine. Some days I didn't know which was worse, the pain from fibromyalgia or the pain from my injuries. What felt like out of nowhere came devastation. and I understood what "disabled" meant.

It's isn't exclusive to being confined to a wheelchair or losing a limb, but rather not being able to perform a function.

Dis–abled. No longer able.

I rolled this word around in my head as my body fought me and started to win. The pain had become stronger than my desire to work. I was unable to stand, unable to groom more than one or two dogs, unable to bend down or lift, unable to focus and perform because of the brain fog and exhaustion. I must have been running on adrenaline until then.

So now what? What do we do when we just can't anymore?

Most people don't have the luxury of staying at home without generating money. Most of us can't get disability assistance. Not everyone has a partner or family that can support them. Unless we're able to find a way to make money from home, or find a job that properly accommodates our disabilities, we fall through the cracks.

It would be so easy to just give up and give in.

But you know what? We are too strong, too resilient, too determined, to do that. Some of the hardest–working people I know are butterflies. That is why it's even more infuriating when one loses their job or gets reprimanded by their boss for something that is beyond their control.

There is a downside to our determination. Because our disease is invisible, and we conceal it so well, most bosses treat us "normally."

We don't expect special treatment, not that we would get it anyway, but losing your job over something that is out of your control is mentally devastating. We've become accustomed to seeing our disabilities as flaws and defects, and accept it when someone else does the same.

People wonder why don't we speak up when we're being fired for being late or unproductive? Because no one cares why we are late or unproductive. Society doesn't see our problems as real and tangible, and that includes employers.

Would it make a difference if we told them we're often late because we're on new medications that make us extremely groggy and still figuring out the best time to take them? Doubtful.

If we had a doctor's note explaining our physical limitations, all that translates to is that we cannot perform our duties.

There is no easy answer. Trust us, we've tried.

That is part of the reason fibromyalgia and chronic pain remain so unbelievable, especially in us young butterflies.

We are trapped in a gray area. Not old enough for the benefits of disability assistance, but too young to be sick.

AGEISM

Ageism is typically a complaint from the older generation, but when you live with chronic pain, it becomes all too real. It's not just our peers who judge us by our age either.

Our very own doctors often refuse certain treatments, medications, and tests solely based on our age. Can you imagine having a medication available to you that could be the difference between being bedridden and functioning normally, then having a doctor withhold it because "you're too young and I want to exhaust every other option first."

Thanks. That's just what we were hoping. Swimming and yoga is a much more suitable treatment plan and I'm sure it will magically make working and parenting a breeze.

The best is when you are trying to explain to an older co–worker or family member what your day–to–day pain is like and you get a response like this, "Oh, honey. You have no idea what real pain is yet!" Of course this statement is almost always accompanied by a belittling laugh that adds insult to our injury. But we smile and nod when we really want to shake that person and scream, "You have no idea what it's like to be so young and feel so old!"

You would think we could at least garner some empathy from our older pain warriors, but more often than not, we get the opposite.

We are perpetually trapped.

We don't look sick enough. We are too young. When really, we have it the worst. We have to work, raise families, run households, care for sick parents, all without proper medications and treatment, without any financial assistance benefits and without any sympathy, even from older fellow butterflies.

Not "looking" sick is more of a curse than a blessing. Yet we still push on, we still hold on to hope and roll with the punches.

ON ACCEPTANCE AND FRIENDSHIP

One of the biggest challenges of having chronic pain is accepting it.

Most of us have been told it was all in our head prior to getting diagnosed, so by the time it's "official", our self–doubt has taken over.

Chronic pain is already devastating and comes with constant changes and adjustments. Many of us become resentful and angry, especially when it comes to friendships and our social life. Stories abound of butterflies mourning the loss of a best friend over their disease. We lose a lot of people along the way, including ourselves.

We have to accept us as we are, accept the realities of our disease, and accept that not everyone is prepared to share our journey.

AFTER MY DIAGNOSIS

At first, I only told a small handful of people when I was diagnosed with fibromyalgia. My parents, my husband, and a close aunt.

It's not like announcing a pregnancy or a diagnosis like cancer, but somewhere in between. Being diagnosed with fibromyalgia doesn't offer any solutions, there is no plan of attack or cure. The diagnosis is more of an affirmation than anything else.

Most of the people I have talked to had symptoms for years, decades even, before getting a diagnosis. When I asked if it changed anything, the response was underwhelming.

The most frequent response was, *"I was just relieved to know it wasn't all in my head."*

I felt the same when, after a decade plus of pain, MRIs, x–rays, blood tests, specialists, and physical therapy, my doctor finally connected the dots. By then, it was more of a "told ya so" moment.

I wasn't a wimp, I wasn't a hypochondriac and I was right!

So now what?

I am on different medication now, but aside from that my life is the same as always. People are just as dismissive as before.

Despite proof from my doctors, people continue to shrug it off as a made–up disease. If they can't see it and they can't imagine it, then it must not be that serious.

When I asked the lovely gals in my fibro group how their diagnosis affected them, the response was heartbreaking. "I felt vindicated and relieved... that I wasn't faking it or 'crazy.'"

How tragic is that statement?

We have struggled in silence for years, decades, with constant doubt from those around us.

"My husband told me for 16 years that it was all in my head," one woman shared with me.

We as fibro patients are in a constant uphill battle. Battling the pain every day is one thing, unending as it is, but the hardest battle for me is the emotional one.

A diagnosis does two things: one, confirms that we are not "crazy", and two, confirms that we are, in fact, going to feel like this for the rest of our lives.

Can you imagine realizing that this will be permanent? And in the midst of your mourning and sadness, you are probably standing there alone. The diagnosis is for the patient and is irrelevant to everyone else.

When I was diagnosed, my husband just shrugged.

Granted, he is the most supportive, helpful person in my day–to–day life, but still it felt heartbreaking. There I was, stunned to find out that not only am I not a hypochondriac, but that my body will forever function this way, and all my husband could do was shrug? Like it was nothing more than a word.

But in a way, that is true. Fibromyalgia is simply a word. Ask anyone who has it and they will probably agree.

We are so used to living this way, and even more used to being disregarded, ignored, and mocked, that we use that word as proof. Fibromyalgia is a diagnosis that says "I am not making this up!"

When someone rolls their eyes at us, we can say "I have fibromyalgia" in defense.

We have to defend ourselves from the sarcasm, from the know–it–alls who like to tell us yoga and sleep will cure us, from the doctors who accuse us of being pill–seekers.

I have heard too many stories of people having to defend themselves from loved ones, husbands, children, employers, and doctors. We are supposed to be reducing our stress, yet we are in a constant state of defense, ready for battle at any moment with our diagnoses as our shield.

A woman in my group said she was depressed after her diagnosis at first, but *"then I decided to pull myself up by my bootstraps and deal with it. I realized that millions of people have chronic illnesses that they live with. And I also decided to be grateful that I finally knew what was wrong with me and that I wasn't just a lazy wimp. It was very validating."*

She nailed it.

A diagnosis validates us but it shouldn't change our lives. It is simply a word to describe everything we go through every day. After all, when we get diagnosed we don't automatically become bedridden. We keep raising our children, going to work, swimming, writing, and so on.

We do what we always do, push ourselves harder than we think is possible every single day.

A diagnosis should empower us to take control of our disease and find ways to live our lives as best we can, it should give us a voice to speak up and be heard and find friends like us, and it should make us realize that we are stronger and more powerful than we could have ever known before diagnosis. And most of all, it should tell you that you matter, your voice counts and that you can keep going.

"YOU'RE SO ANTI–SOCIAL!"

I used to function like a normal person. Go out to bars, stay up till 3 a.m., walk around downtown, and shop for hours. And by "used to", I mean up until last year.

I'm 33, still very young considering the nature of my disease, and most of my peers still spend their weekends out all night. They celebrate birthdays at clubs and function at work on five hours of sleep.

Over the past year, I have found myself having to decline these invites more and more. Between working a very physically demanding job for forty hours a week, where I also talk 8 hours straight,, raising two small children, and dealing with fibromyalgia and social anxiety, those activities are not feasible for me anymore.

At first I felt tremendous guilt. I thought I didn't have an actual reason for not wanting to go, so I would say "I'm tired" or "I don't feel good."

I tried to think of every excuse I could to decline any and all invites. I used my kids as an excuse a lot more than I'd like to admit.

I assumed my friends would take it personally and accuse me of being lazy. They did at first give me some shit for it. "Oh just suck it up and come." So I would. Then by 11 p.m., my body would be screaming at me to go to bed. I'd wince through the pain and fatigue, sipping my beer that I knew I would regret later. By then one or two drinks left me feeling like I had the flu for the next couple days.

When I got my diagnosis, I felt such relief. No longer did I have to make excuses. My absence was now justified. My friends no longer prodded at me when I said I didn't feel like doing something. It felt so liberating to have such understanding friends. The pressure was off.

But then, little by little, the invites became few and far between. I started feeling left out as I would browse through my Facebook feed filled with pictures of my friends having a blast out past 10 p.m.

I would send them texts asking why I wasn't included or if they were mad at me.

They explained that they knew I wouldn't want to come. Not in a mean way, but an understanding way.

Like okay, Joanna. You're off the hook.

At first I wasn't sure how I felt about this. It dawned on me that the voice in my head was being naïve when it said "I am going to turn down all your invites but I still want you to invite me every time!"

I had to let go of the old me, and learn to make decisions that were right for me. I'm a lot happier for it too.

My friends know that they are more than welcome to drop by my house anytime they wish and I'm always up for coffee and conversation from the comfort of my couch. They know they can text me and I will always answer quickly and wholeheartedly.

I'm not a bad friend, I'm just a friend with fibromyalgia. All I can do is be the best friend possible with what resources I have.

My truest of friends wouldn't want me doing things detrimental to my well–being anyway, so I look at it like a friend–filter.

Call me anti–social, I don't care. For me, my phone and computer are my lifeline. I can interact, socialize, write, read, and chat to my heart's content while wrapped up in my heating pad.

Invite me out for a nice dinner party and I am likely to accept, as long as I can be home by 11 p.m. I love nothing more than to host a get–together at my casa, too. Every year we host a huge Christmas Eve party.

I hear things like, "Don't you get bored always being at home?" and "You need to get out more!" on repeat and I just smile. To be honest, there is nowhere else I would rather be. My body feels the best at home.

I am the "anti–social mom" and I'm pretty darn content with it.

NORMAL FRIENDS

"Keep inviting me! I really want to come! I really really really do! I may say "No" most of the time, but the few times I am able to say yes mean the world to me. It takes a lot for me to go out and I usually need a lot of rest after. Don't forget about me just because I'm sick. I still want to be a part of your life." — *Gloria L.*

Once in a while, we might find someone "normal" who not only believes us, but voluntarily talks to and listens to us talk about our disease. I call this the "people jackpot." Most of the butterflies I know have maybe one or two healthy people in their lives who show empathy.

I don't know why it's so hard for healthy people to be friends with someone who is chronically ill. And it's not limited to those of us with chronic pain.

Depression, anxiety, bipolar, etc., are avoided at all costs in conversation. This is why invisible illnesses are so isolating, healthy people don't understand or don't want to understand. Are they scared? Do they not want to admit that their friend is sick? Do they just not want to deal with it? I honestly don't know because they've all slipped away and I never got to ask.

We miss you.

We blame ourselves for the demise of our relationships. We don't want you to have to deal with our disease, but if you want to have a friendship, you will have to make room for our dark passenger. No, we probably won't make it to the nightclub, we might cancel dinner a few times a month, and shopping just isn't happening.

But we can listen to you. We can support and love you. We can still laugh and cry with you. We can text all day and finish our conversations on the couch all night. We're the perfect friend, we have nothing else to do but be there for you!

"Validation is what I crave most. I rarely ever feel like anyone cares enough to try and understand and more often than not they make me feel like my pain is exaggerated by me or even made up for attention. I hear things like "are you ever not sick?" or "does any part of your body NOT hurt?" or "don't you get tired of hearing yourself complain?" That's why we shut down and quit talking about our pain to the people we love. It hurts because they're supposed to love us too!" — Anonymous

BODY ENVY

Just as our friends and family have to accept that our bodies just don't work anymore, we have to accept that their bodies do. I catch myself watching co-workers doing the exact same thing as me and I wonder "How can she just do that? I wonder what it's like to do this with no pain?"

Most of us can't remember what it's like to be pain–free.

We have bad days and we have "badder" days. Even with medications and treatments, we are lucky if we get our pain down to a 2. Your worst day is a normal day for us.

Some of us have been sick since childhood and have no recollection of ever being without pain.

As we watch our friends and family do all the things we can't, not without pain, we begin to compare bodies. This magnifies our anger and leads us to hate our bodies even more.

Why can't we just be normal? Why me?

We would give anything to trade bodies with you, even for a day.

But instead of resenting our bodies, we need to see how incredible we are. We do everything we can, everything "normal" people are doing, but we're doing it with crippling pain and fatigue and a smile on our face.

How extraordinary is that?

So next time you find yourself comparing your sick body to someone else's, don't forget just how powerful and strong your body is!

ON DOCTORS AND TREATMENTS

"It took me forever to get anything prescribed for the pain. The minute you see a doctor for pain, they assume that you are just med–seeking and have no actual reason to need the medication." — Taylor S.

More and more doctors are implementing a "pain acceptance" method of "treatment" for chronic pain patients.

This method avoids the use of opioids, and includes alternatives like physical therapy, yoga, etc. You know, those things many of us have tried without success. According to Dr. Jane Ballantyne, the doctor who first introduced this idea in 2015, doctors and patients should acknowledge that the pain will never be at a zero and we should just accept and live with our pain.

Medically sound, indeed.

Most people who live with chronic pain don't believe it will ever get to a zero, but we do believe that we have the right to adequate treatment and care from our doctors. Their responsibility is to help us find a way to minimize the pain as much as possible. Telling us to deal with it and try yoga sure sounds a lot like they're giving up on us.

Maybe it's the doctors, and our government, who need to practice "pain acceptance."

I accept that my pain will never go away, never be anywhere near a zero, and never will there exist a magic pill or exercise that will fix it.

I accept that when my doctor is doing everything he can to help me maintain the best quality of life possible, I will do the same. But if my doctor cannot accept the fact that I have a disease that causes me perpetual pain, nor accept the fact that opioid medications are often the most effective and practical pain management option, then maybe that doctor shouldn't be treating patients with pain.

It seems that doctors and our government have washed their hands of us chronic pain patients.

Would a doctor refuse someone the medication for their illness? No, because the doctor knows how dangerous that could be for the patient's well–being. So why is it acceptable for them to do that to us?

We accept our pain, we accept that opioids and other medications have risks like anything else, and we accept responsibility for our part in our treatment.

When will everyone else accept it?

THE PEOPLE OR THE DATA

While many doctors accuse us of "doctor shopping" like it's a bad thing, the truth is we are. We are shopping for a doctor who listens to us, who sees us.

The problem is, we've become jaded. Many of us have given up completely and don't bother with a doctor, and that can wind up pretty dangerous. I don't know how many people I've talked to who ignored a pain for too long and wound up in the hospital with pancreatitis or some other serious problem.

We ignore it, we self–medicate, and we go without treatments, all to avoid one more crappy doctor.

I once went to an orthopedic urgent care at a really "good" hospital. I brought all my bloodwork and medical history, and was prepared to get help for a shoulder injury. As the doctor read through my file, I clenched my body up, nervously sputtering out symptoms and thoughts as he took inventory.

"Ah. Fibromyalgia. I see," he said sternly, slapping my file closed. He left the room for a few minutes and returned with a print out that listed three doctors names. "Here is a list of doctors who believe in this sort of stuff. I can't help you." He started to leave the room and my eyes welled up with tears.

"But, but, what about my— " I started desperately.

"Take some ibuprofen. I don't know what to tell you." And with that, he left.

Mind you, he had just read in my bloodwork that I could not take NSAIDs because of my kidneys.

After he left, I had a complete breakdown. I sobbed so hard two nurses came running in. They comforted me awkwardly and walked me out of the office. I have never had a public breakdown, but I have also never been treated so poorly by a doctor in my life.

Later, after filing a complaint with the administration, I discovered via Yelp that this doctor was known for this dismissive, rude behavior. So, why is he still practicing?

Why is this hospital letting him run an urgent care center for people in pain?

And why isn't my pain important?

My story is not uncommon.

If you ask anyone with chronic pain, they could give you five more stories like mine, especially in urgent care and the emergency room.

I call it the "doctor–go–round."

Within my first year of diagnosis, I saw nine doctors. General practitioners, specialists, you name it. They passed me off to one another, threw some meds at me, and shrugged me off.

There is nothing worse than living in the hell of chronic pain and being denied not only treatment, but respect.

The problem is doctors look at data, not people.

Even though we are sitting right in front of them, describing our pain and symptoms, telling them what we need, the data holds more weight. Why is it that doctors say that opioids don't work for chronic pain? Is it because there are thousands of chronic pain patients saying "my opioids don't help"?

Hint, there isn't.

Is it because there is extensive, solid research proving this?

No. No, there isn't that either.

Not only is there virtually no research on long–term efficacy of opioids on chronic pain, but there are probably millions of chronic pain patients who depend on opioid medications just to get up and go to work every day. Yes, there are downsides to opioid medications, but for those of us with chronic pain, they don't get us "high", they get us "normal."

Yet doctors, scientists and even politicians still scream, until they are blue in the face, that opioids are useless.

Why aren't patients factored in? Why aren't our real–life stories part of their research? Why is it that my friend, who took her opioids as prescribed, responsibly, for over twelve years, was told she could no longer have them because they weren't working.

She was forcibly withdrawn from her medication and left with no other treatment in its place despite having a relatively normal life thanks to that very medication. Her doctor made his decision due to data, not his patient.

One gal in my support group summed it up perfectly: "You know medicine, I know my body... Finding good doctors isn't easy and when you're chronically ill, you need even better ones!"

I trust my doctor to oversee and guide my treatment and care, not dictate which meds are working for me or not. I am an adult, and I know my body, and I know what it is doing and how it is responding.

Listen to me.

On the flipside, I've had doctors shove medications down my throat despite my protests. I had one doctor who was determined to make one particular medication work for me. I trusted him, so I tried it.

The side effects were terrifying. I hallucinated, I couldn't sleep, couldn't eat, I became paranoid and believed someone was coming to take my kids in the night. When I informed him, he decided to change up the dosage.

Thanks. Great.

A change in the dosage, but no change in side effects.

I did my own research, most of us have to, and discovered a massive list of frightening side effects, including suicide and death, for the medication.

When I spoke with him again, he changed my dosage. I smiled and nodded, trying to keep my disbelief hidden, and went home and promptly threw the medication into the trash.

Never again.

TRUST

How much do you trust your doctor? Do you trust your life with him? Because you should. Because that is their job, to care for your health, safety and well-being. But doctors are making it increasingly difficult to trust them.

Butterflies often wonder when and if he will give up on us and "fire" us. Or when he will cut off our medications out of fear. Or if he even believes us. Have you ever gone to the doctor and been told you're making it up?

We have. A lot.

We have been misdiagnosed more times than we can even count.

Would you trust your doctor after he dismissed something as part of your chronic illness, only to later discover it was cancer? True story, sadly, but I'll have to save that for another book.

Or gone to the emergency room, desperate for help, only to be turned away because they don't treat chronic illness, wind up in an ambulance a few hours later? Also a true story.

Our doctors don't trust us to begin with.

Many believe our disease is psychological and treat us accordingly.

"Think the pain away."

"Take your antidepressants."

"Meditate."

No, doc. Our pain is real. But they don't trust something they can't see proof of. There is no test for chronic pain. It doesn't show up on an x–ray. And our testimony doesn't count, either.

Here we have a cycle.

Doctor doesn't trust us, doctor misdiagnoses, wrongly–medicates us, or hands us off, we lose trust in doctors, and we give up. And when we give up, when we lose that trust, we start ignoring our symptoms. We try and trudge on without a treatment plan, without relief, without hope.

One fellow butterfly told me that she fell and hurt her ankle once. The pain was severe, but she didn't go to the doctor because she believed her doctor would shrug it off as "just part of your fibro." So she limped around for days, which turned into weeks, until finally her ankle was so swollen and distorted, she was forced to go to the emergency room.

Turns out it was broken in multiple spots and she required surgery immediately.

This is why trust is vital. We need to know that our doctors believe us and will do everything they swore to do, help us the best they can with the best care and treatment available.

When we don't trust, we ignore pain, we ignore symptoms and put ourselves in dangerous situations because of it. Our tolerance to pain is already skewed. What might feel like an eight to a normal person is probably an average day for one of us. This means that if we fracture something, we probably wouldn't even notice.

Another woman in my group ignored a new pain and woke up in the hospital with a burst appendix.

After losing the trust of our doctors, we eventually lose trust in ourselves and our bodies. That's when we stop taking care of ourselves, stop trying and let go of hope.

That's when the depression sets in and chronic pain gets dangerous.

BUT HAVE YOU TRIED TURMERIC?

Not only do we have to deal with doctors using us as guinea pigs by guessing 90% of our treatments and care, we get more unsolicited advice than you can imagine from family, friends, hair stylists, and, of course, the people of the internet.

"You're only as healthy as you make up your mind to be. At least you don't have cancer. You don't have a brain tumor. You're not in a wheelchair. Stop acting like you're sick."

Yes, that is an actual statement from the father of a fibromyalgia patient.

I'm not sure why the world thinks that people with chronic pain are so unbelievable. We believe people with heart conditions, diabetes, arthritis, etc. We don't debate taking away their meds. We don't pretend to understand what they are dealing with and tell them how to manage their disease.

And we certainly don't judge them.

What is it about fibromyalgia that gives people license to comment on our weight, for instance? If fibromyalgia is caused by obesity, then how do you explain all the svelte sufferers out there?

If it's dietary, then why do the uber–healthy eaters get stuck with it? One of my favorites that we hear all–too–often is that we're just depressed. This is a theory widely used by doctors, too. We are being prescribed antidepressants now in lieu of pain medications, which ultimately means the doc is telling us this is all in our head.

The amount of fibromyalgia "experts" in the world is astounding.

It's hard to believe that with so much knowledge out there, we still don't know the cause or cure.

Actually, we don't even know how to manage it.

Doctors and patients spend lifetimes doing trial and error with various medications and treatments. Yet it's the social media "doctors" who baffle me the most. People seem to think they know better than us because they have a friend who...

When I first began this painful journey, I lived completely natural. I ate a 90/10 vegan whole–foods diet, worked out daily, took herbs and supplements, and considered it a bad day when I had to take ibuprofen.

Now I realize how minimal my symptoms were back then.

Now I have a mixed regimen of treatments. I still take my supplements, eat clean, practice self–care, walk, etc., but I also take prescription medications and I don't have to defend my choices.

Too often people feel justified in judging us for taking prescription medications.

"You know that fill–in–the–blank is just going to make it worse, right?"

You know what? Let me worry about that.

I am doing the best I can and making informed decisions for me. Unless you are living in my body, you have no right to dictate how I manage my disease.

Do you think I like depending on medications to function? I don't.

But I would rather use these medications that allow me to be as close to normal as possible than suffer and remain bedridden. Because that's the other option.

You don't know how much yoga, how many diets, how many supplements, acupuncture, meditation, therapy, and coconut oil I have tried before finally giving in to "Big Pharma".

Please keep your judgment and shaming to yourself.

We are our own worst enemy as it is and don't need any help with feeling bad. We have to find what works for each of us individually and welcome your thoughts and ideas, but skip the condescending lecture and offer something with more sympathy.

For example; instead of the snide comment a few paragraphs up, say something like *"I've heard that that medication might have some dangerous side effects. I just wanted you to know because I care about your well–being."*

Believe me, the outcome will be much better for everyone. You can still bring ideas to the table, but don't shove them down our throat.

"To the people who tell me I should come off the prescriptions that allow me to function; does that mean I should stop asthma inhalers? Or a diabetic should stop insulin? It really winds me up, this media–fuelled misconception that taking pain meds is the same as being a drug addict. I don't take them to escape reality, I take them to lead a productive life. To liken that to being a junkie is offensive, dismissive, and cruel." — Jeannie M.

THE HIDDEN TRUTH

There is a dark side to fibromyalgia and chronic pain. The time we spend with our dark passenger overtakes us.

Sometimes it's just for a day, sometimes it's forever, but when we turn off our smile and collapse under the weight of this disease, we find ourselves in a dark, desperate place. We think things we wouldn't dare admit to "normal" people.

Things that are so taboo we become afraid of ourselves.

As my little support group grew in strength, I noticed more and more people confessing their hidden truths. I posted a photo of myself completely vulnerable, at the deepest point of despair. I felt silly for having taken a photo of myself like that, but I did it anyway.

I had fallen on the stairs and couldn't get up. All I could do was cry. My dog came to my rescue and furiously licked my tears away, nudging my face with his, pushing his body against mine, trying desperately to comfort me.

The picture was embarrassing, but I was so sick of putting on a mask and just wanted someone, anyone to see me. To see my pain, my exhaustion, my face swollen from medication, my aloneness. To me, this moment was the most real and raw and I needed to tell someone.

The most beautiful thing happened.

People responded by posting their own hidden truth photos. Dozens of people like me, my friends, alone and in pain. I wasn't the only one who had needed to capture their darkest, realest moments.

Here we were in all our "ugly" glory, showing that at the end of the day, we are alone with our dark passenger. These were the faces of fibromyalgia, of neverending pain.

But these were also the faces of strength, perseverance, endurance, sacrifice, and hope.

Pain, fatigue, and a seemingly endless list of physical symptoms aren't the only battles we face.

There are psychological and emotional symptoms of chronic pain that you won't find on WebMD. While depression and anxiety are so common in patients that they are listed as actual symptoms, there is no explanation as to why.

Normal people have a hard time making the connection between depression and pain, and some people even blame our chronic pain on our depression.

It's actually the other way around.

Pushing through pain, we can do. We do it every day. But pushing through all of the mental struggles can be more damaging than the pain.

While it's easy to tell someone you're tired or you're hurting, telling someone you feel alone and hopeless is terrifying. We go from warrior to vulnerable and feel shame and guilt. Not only is our pain invisible, but so is our suffering, and we keep it that way to avoid judgment or worse.

This is our hidden truth.

THE "S" WORD

"My pain is an aching all over my body that I can't escape or make it stop even for a moment. My muscles and joints feel torn and inflamed. It is exhausting. I often think how easy it would be to just make it stop, escape my torturous body. But I have my son that needs me — I have to live with this pain for the rest of my days. The loss of hope for relief is the most crushing thing." — Sarah C. G.

We used to be afraid of the "S" word. If someone used it, all hell would break loose. People would panic, lose their minds with fear. After a while, after we became comfortable with one another, we began using the "S" word openly and honestly.

Sometimes, I want to die.

Sometimes, suicide feels like my only option.

Sometimes, I wish the pain would just end.

That doesn't mean we are suicidal. It's not a threat and it's certainly not a cry for attention. It's a part of our disease. It is a side effect of never ending pain and fatigue. Doctors tell us our pain is actually depression.

Well, doc, if you experienced pain and fatigue and the rest of the symptoms we do every single day with no relief, I bet you'd be a bit depressed, too.

"Sometimes, the want to make it stop gets so bad. Not because I want to die, no, it's because it hurts too much to live. But I can't do that. Not to my kids. So I pull it together and drive my pain deeper." — Sarah R.

The magical thing about us butterflies is our ability to empathize. If I mention wanting to die to my husband or friends, I'm met with a gasp and "Oh, don't say that!" But my people get it. We know exactly what it means.

It means we are tired. Tired of the pain, the isolation, the shame and guilt. It means we are getting weary and need a break. It means we just need to reach out and find someone who understands.

A person can only live with such intense, incessant, intractable pain and emotional suffering for so long before they become desperate for relief. But relief eventually seems like a fairytale when, after trying all the medications, therapies and treatments from a carousel of doctors and specialists, our symptoms remain.

Remember the worst pain you've ever felt? Maybe a car accident or broken bones?

Now imagine feeling that every day for the rest of your life. Then imagine that no one believes you so no one will help you.

The pain keeps you from participating in life and you watch friends and family carry on, pain–free, without you. Would you be a ball of sunshine?

So when we talk about suicide, we aren't talking about ending our life. We are talking about ending our pain and suffering. There is a difference.

Listen to us, be there for us and, most of all, let us speak.

ISOLATION

There are a lot of reasons we end up using the "S" word, and loneliness is one of them. In the early stages of our disease, we can still function relatively well. We go out dancing, to dinner, stay up late, work overtime. Eventually, for most people, it progresses.

It progresses to the point where we start missing out on birthday parties and holidays. Then we become maxed out at twenty work hours and start getting in trouble for missing work and underperforming. We're home more. In bed more. Our partner starts getting frustrated with our lack of energy and participation in life and the relationship. We break–up. Our friends stop inviting us out because they assume we won't come anyway. Family stops visiting because they don't know what to do with us.

Ultimately, the majority of our life is spent alone.

Isolation obviously leads to depression. Before social media, finding others with chronic pain wasn't easy, especially because it's hard to get out, and if you do, no one likes to talk about it. I often wonder how many lives have been saved because of support online. I have reached out in my darkest hours and found strangers pulling me back, more than people in "real life."

Without my support group, I would truly be alone with my pain. I didn't know anyone with fibromyalgia when I was first diagnosed and it was frightening. I had so many questions that my healthy doctor couldn't answer; questions only a fellow butterfly would understand, like if a symptom is normal or home remedies that actually help.

One of the most common phrases I see in my support group is; "I am so relieved –I thought it was just me!" Discovering that you are not alone, that everything you think and feel is actually normal, is infinitely comforting. Describing the relief would be impossible.

We know how to push through pain. We can barrel through fatigue. But the isolation will suck the life right out of you. The isolation will suck out any inkling of hope and joy, leaving you wondering why you should even bother fighting anymore.

NOT GUILTY

"If you're feeling annoyed that my chronic pain has inconvenienced you, affected your plans, or otherwise caused you frustration, then consider what my chronic pain has done to me. Reacting to my pain because of its impact on you amplifies the feelings of guilt and shame, which in turn amplifies the pain." — Nicole A.

I've mentioned guilt a few times in this book and now I'm going to address it. You might wonder what guilt has to do with chronic pain, but any of us will tell you it is an overwhelmingly present symptom. We feel like bad parents, bad spouses, bad children, bad employees, bad friends, bad people.

Why are we bad?

Because we let everyone down. We fail. We can't. Guilt is just another part of our dark passenger.

Looking into your sweet child's face and telling them "no, we can't", for the hundredth time and seeing the look of disappointment is like a knife to the gut. Or seeing the frustration in your partner's eyes when you decline intimacy again. Being unable to care for your ailing parent and watching a hired nurse do it instead. These are all things that lead to one feeling – guilt.

We want so much to be "normal". Letting people down every day gets increasingly frustrating. But again, we keep the guilt to ourselves. We apologize relentlessly. It becomes compulsive, even.

It sounds silly to apologize for things beyond our control. People tell us not to feel bad and that it's not our fault, but the problem is we've been told our pain isn't real, or our pain can be cured if we just do this or change that, or that our pain is emotional. So now we feel like our pain is our fault and become angry and frustrated with our own bodies.

We know you mean well when you tell us that we can cure our fibromyalgia by thinking positively and doing yoga, but it just adds to the stress and guilt. It makes us think "Gee, I've done those things and they didn't work. I'm failing at that, too." We are made to feel guilty a hundred times a day, albeit unintentionally.

Letting people down means letting yourself down. We feel shame for not doing yoga. We feel shame for taking medication. We feel guilt for not doing the dishes. We feel guilt for not being able to get out of bed. It's endless and it swallows us whole.

But why should we feel guilty? It's not our fault. It really isn't. That's something we all need to learn and accept. Stop allowing guilt and shame to eat you alive. We didn't ask for this and we do our best every day. We are not the ones who should feel guilty. Those who don't even try to understand, those who shame us, who abandon us, those are the ones who should feel bad.

"I'M FINE."

Our two favorite words, and our biggest lie. You see, if we answered honestly, you wouldn't like it. Not only that, but there would likely never be a time when we would be "fine." There are so many reasons behind this answer.

"I feel like complete hell but I am sick of saying it."

"I am just going to pretend like everything's fine to mask my pain."

"I don't feel like admitting to how I'm really feeling."

"I feel horrible, but you wouldn't understand."

"You wouldn't believe me anyway."

"I don't want to be a whiner or complainer."

We say we're fine to spare either your feelings or ours. We are not fine. We are exhausted and hurting. We are depressed and anxious. We also cannot stand to deal with one more inane response. Here's what happens if we answer honestly: "Well, I'm really struggling right now. My pain is overwhelming."

"That's too bad. My back has been pretty achy lately, too."

Diminishing our pain and symptoms makes us feel like crap.

"You know, maybe you should start going to the gym! Movement always helps."

No, no. That's not how this works.

"I know what you mean."

Oh, you do? I didn't know you were magically diagnosed with fibromyalgia overnight.

I don't mean to be snarky, but we get responses like this almost every time, so we lie. We pretend. We grin and bear it. "How are you doing?" is a loaded question for us. Every time we talk about our disease, we become vulnerable to insult and condescending remarks. It is easier and safer to pretend like we're fine.

But maybe we need to stop. Maybe it's time to brace ourselves and tell our truth. If we continue telling people we're fine, we can't expect people's' perception of chronic pain to change. It's not whining, it's not complaining and if someone doesn't understand, try and make them.

OUR PLEA

"We are heroes for enduring... every day and despite our illness try to live as much of a normal life as possible. Everything we do in life is so much harder, and yet we do so much anyway. We have grit and we had to learn to be resilient to not give up despite our illness. There's a lot that healthy people can learn from us because of this." — Chana K.

One good thing about chronic pain is that it gives you perspective. We take pleasure in seemingly small things like a new pillow or a medication that works.

We don't worry about frivolous things which in turn makes us grateful in general. A kind word, a good TV show, a night of sleep. We understand the value of these small joys. We don't want much, honestly, which made me wonder – what do butterflies want? Deep down, we must want more than a good heating blanket and a nice doctor, so what is it?

To be seen and heard.

That's it. That's all we want. To be acknowledged and understood. To go a day without someone dismissing our pain, our loneliness, our needs.

This brought me to another question.

If you could say one thing to "normal" people, what would it be? I asked my support group to pretend they had the attention of all the "normal" people in the world (and that they were actually listening) and all of the responses could be put into at least one of three categories.

If you are one of the "normal" people I refer to, and you have made it to the end of this book, I want to share with you the three pleas and I want you to hear us. I mean really, truly hear us.

BELIEVE US

"I know it's difficult to understand something you can't experience yourself, I don't expect you to. Just believe me when I say I'm in pain, or I'm so tired I can barely move. I feel ashamed of myself enough as it is so I don't need you to shame me for not doing 'enough.'" — Aurora G.

Why is it so unbelievable? What is it about pain that makes people so skeptical? Do people honestly believe that we would make something like this up? Yes, we have a fake disease just to garner attention and sympathy. Only, we rarely receive either of those things, let alone proper care and treatment. It's a real blast missing out on life and being judged and dismissed day in and day out. If we were going to fake a disease for attention, don't you think we would choose something believable?

"I'm not faking this and my symptoms are real and more severe than they can imagine. Why would I make up a debilitating illness, when all I want in this life is to be healthy?" — Taylor S.

"This disease is real, this pain is real. If I could have one wish, it wouldn't be money, it would be my health back." — Sebana A.

DON'T JUDGE US

"Just because I am sitting up, smiling and keeping up your conversation, and kept some food down today does not mean that I feel how I appear. We learned not to judge a book by its cover, why can't we apply that to other beings?" — Caitlin G.

We know when we're being judged. The looks we get when we're taking our meds, the eye–rolling when we are struggling to work, and, of course, the comments. I'm not sure why people feel so entitled to make hurtful comments toward us.

"Dont judge what you don't want nor have tried to understand!" — Jennifer W.

We are so hard on ourselves as it is. We have to cope not only with our symptoms, but with the guilt, anger, frustration and hopelessness of our condition.

Judgment hurts. A lot. This is why we shut down.

We stop talking about our pain, our sadness, our feelings, because we live in fear of being judged. Even the people who are supposed to love us unconditionally are guilty of this. People don't judge people with "visible" illnesses, so why is it OK to do to us? Why is it ok to call us lazy, or to lecture us on the "dangers" of our medications and treatments?

"Don't judge us. If you do, please don't spread your wrong assumptions to others. It's hard enough feeling bad about what we've had to give up with those we love because of this illness, we don't need extra grief…" — Rena J.

WE'RE DOING OUR BEST

"I am doing my best, not just despite my sickness, but to live with my sicknesses. That my illnesses are a part of me, and they're not going away. But there are so many other amazing parts of me: and, honestly, my illnesses have brought out the best in me, even though I wouldn't wish them on my worst enemy. They have brought out a strength and resilience in me that I never imagined I would possess. They have taught me I can overcome and get through anything." — Kat G.

We live in a world full of expectations. Socially, economically, physically, mentally, we are all supposed to be a certain way.

This is stressful for even the healthiest of people, so imagine what the struggle is like for us. Taking a shower can be a debilitating event, and somehow we are supposed to have a successful career, raise a family, be physically fit, etc?

Our best is different from "the" best. And our best is enough. It may seem to you that we are not trying or that we are giving up and giving in to our illness, but it's quite the opposite. We do everything you do, but we have to do it with pain, fatigue, and many other debilitating issues, not to mention all the negativity from people around us.

We have to pick and choose what we spend our energy on, so while you think we're being lazy because our laundry is piling up, it's because we spend the night before at a friend's birthday party and paid for it with our body the next day.

"What I live with is my normal, you may not get it and you may think I'm over dramatic but I do the best I can and I figure it out as I go. I'm just as capable to handle anything as anyone else it just might take me longer sometimes." — Mary Elizabeth H.

Please, try and put yourself in our place and show us kindness and empathy. We do so much to please everyone around us, to meet the expectations society puts on us, to not let anyone down. The weight of it is crushing, yet we persevere not for our sake, but for yours. Remember that.

"I wish people understood that we are trying our best. That every day is a new struggle. Yet we face it head on because we know that there is no choice. We either fight back or get consumed by this awful disease that is incurable. That we try our best but we realize that we don't live up to your standards. We would just like to be accepted for who we are and loved just the same if not more." — Krista G.

TO THE BUTTERFLIES

I want to say something to you, butterflies. I need you to do three things:

1. DON'T APOLOGIZE

Butterflies tend to apologize compulsively and especially when there is no reason for it. Don't be sorry for taking your medications, your treatment is just as valuable as anyone else's. Don't be sorry for your messy house, it doesn't mean you're lazy, it means you were prioritizing your energy.

Do not apologize for skipping the birthday party, for leaving work early, for sleeping late. You do your best and your best is enough. Never feel bad for doing enough.

2. SPEAK UP

The silence is killing us. We have been trained to keep our mouths shut, to bury our feelings, to cover up our disease and symptoms. We will never be understood, respected or treated properly if we let the world speak for us.

Tell your story. Be honest about your symptoms. Ask for help.

Every time someone makes a negative comment, educate them. Words are powerful, and if we all speak up, we will make a difference. Your words can inspire someone else to speak up for themselves. Your words can transform people. Don't hide anymore, butterflies. Your pain is real, your disease is real, and you deserve to be heard.

3. LOVE YOURSELF

We spend so much time and energy trying to please the world around us, self–care gets cast by the wayside. We don't feel that we deserve love, we don't deserve care, and that we are such terrible people because we are sick that we have to pay for it by sacrificing ourselves. But these are lies stemming from guilt, and guilt is false.

Loving yourself is the most vital part of getting through this life with chronic pain. You deserve it. Write yourself notes on your mirror, read motivational books, cut toxic people out of your life, indulge in your favorite ice cream, do whatever the hell it takes to love yourself.

I know we pour all of our love into our friends, families, careers, etc. But we seem to forget the one person who needs love the most. We must stop depriving ourselves, stop hurting ourselves and punishing ourselves.

FINAL THOUGHTS

You are not alone. There are people here just like you who truly know your struggles, who understand you to the core, who feel the weight of their dark passenger always present. Reach out and find someone, anyone, who will listen. Whether you find a support group, or a healthy friend, or your family, just reach. You don't have to endure this by yourself. We are here, ready to listen and support you.

You are worthy. You are good. You are doing your best and that's all anyone can ask. Keep going, keep pushing, and don't lose hope. Do whatever it is you need to to cope and make it through. Whether it's art, writing, music, advocacy, starting a support group or joining one, whatever it takes to cope.

Your pain is valid. You are a person just like everyone else, and you deserve love, care and treatment. If you fall, there are people ready to lift you up. Don't be afraid to be yourself, to express your pain and to need help.

It will always be a struggle, but you don't have to go through it alone.

ABOUT THE AUTHOR

Joanna has been writing for over 20 years and has been published on multiple blog sites in addition to publishing her first book, Confessions of Butterflies.

Though her favorite things include dogs, music and her kids, she writes about living with chronic pain. She shares her experiences with humor and honesty, hoping to connect the chronic pain community.

27076291R00043

Made in the USA
Columbia, SC
18 September 2018